COMPLETE PALAEOLITHIC DIET FOR BEGINNERS

PERMITTED AND BENEFICIAL FOODS, FORBIDDEN FOOD, LEARN THE BASICS AND HISTORY OF THIS STYLE OF FEEDING

Jessy M. Brown

Table of Contents

Introduction: A new reality

Like it or not, the health of our society is bad and getting worse.

As technology continues to develop, so does convenience, and ordering food is literally as simple as pushing a button. The days when you had to find your own food, let alone drive to a restaurant for dinner, are long gone.

Cooking dinner seems less and less appealing when compared to the comforts of food and choices between diners, catering services, fast food and take-away.

According to the Academy of Nutrition

and Dietetics, diabetes is now the seventh leading cause of death in the United States alone.

Type 2 diabetes has been on the rise due to poor lifestyle choices, such as too much unhealthy food and too little exercise. "Globesity," a term coined by the World Health Organization to describe the global obesity epidemic, is also another problem. These numbers continue to rise, as do health problems and associated diseases.

As governments and local communities begin to feel the impact of obesity, diabetes, hypertension, etc. due to poor lifestyle choices, awareness increases.

Cheap and processed foods are so easy to come by and overwhelm supermarket shelves. Throw away desk jobs, long trips or displacements and electronics in the mix, and we do a lot of sitting around and very little to burn processed food.

Americans spent about 25 percent of their net income on food ninety years ago, according to a study by RAND on why Americans are so fat. Currently, we spend less than 1 billion euros on construction.

ten percent of that income in food. But we're certainly not eating less, we're eating more, more unhealthy and cheaper.

But maybe we're finally seeing a turning point. In the last three quarters, McDonalds has experienced an overall decline of around 3.3% in sales, which may be indicative of lower consumption of fast food.

With the media covering the obesity epidemic and health and quality of life plummeting, some people are beginning to see the light. Documentaries such as Fed Up are exposing the concerns of food manufacturers who rely only on benefits and not health, and how added sugar is found in more than 80% of supermarket foods.

We may be a long way from returning to "the good old days," where dinner was made with what was in the garden and processed foods were almost unknown. But the best thing we can do is to learn why healthy choices are the best choices for long-term health and quality of life.

As technology develops, our options will continue to grow. By making wise, we can help combat and curb this growing epidemic.

So today I want to give you a quick overview for beginners of one of the best choices you can make regarding overall health and a natural way to eat. The Paleo Diet...Don't worry if you don't know what it is, in the coming moments you will discover why it has been one of the most commented diets of recent times.

Let's dive into...

What the Paleolithic Diet Really Is

If you don't know what the Paleo diet is or haven't heard of it before, don't worry, in this first chapter we will explore exactly what this way of eating is all about.

In its essence, Paleo is much more of a lifestyle than a diet. A Paleo lifestyle consists of eating real, whole and natural foods and avoiding all processed foods.

The modern diet is exactly that, it's modern. Humans ate Paleo-style from the beginning of time before the agricultural revolution began, where we began to eat grains and sugar-based foods, as well as processed foods.

The idea behind Paleo is to eliminate those processed foods, chemicals, vegetable oils and other new additions to the modern diet that can be detrimental to our lifestyle, from how we move to our energy levels to how we feel every day.

During all those years we ate Paleo, humans were hunters and gatherers. They ate meat and fruit like berries when they were in season. Which also meant they moved around a lot and were very active. They needed to be strong and fit to survive. Their bodies were conditioned to use fat efficiently as fuel and energy, not carbohydrates.

Over time, agriculture emerged and the human diet changed drastically.

The Agricultural Revolution occurred about 10,000 years ago and introduced grains, such as wheat and bread, into our diet.

Today's modern diet contains things like significant amounts of gluten. Gluten was non-existent in the Paleolithic. Things like wheat, rye, many cereals and barley contain gluten. It has been recognized that gluten causes inflammation in the intestine and has been given widespread attention through celebrities like Kelly Ripa, who have stopped taking gluten.

It has also been theorized (not proven) that gluten may play a role in increasing the risk of some types of cancer, as well as heart disease.

Another ingredient in the modern diet that is related to possible health problems is that of lectins. The lectins are present in the grains. They cause wear on our gastrointestinal tract, which makes it very difficult to heal.

Let's not forget the sugar. Sugar is everywhere and everywhere today. Sugar has to be burned, but another aspect of modern times is people's sedentary lifestyle.

Everybody sits down. They sit at work, they sit on the couch to watch TV, they sit on their computers, they sit down to check social media and text messages on their smartphones. People do not move as before and therefore do not burn calories as before. This becomes a big problem when talking about sugar consumption.

In the Palaeolithic, humans were thin, strong and fit. They moved, almost all day, every day. They didn't grow or cultivate crops. As I mentioned earlier, they hunted and gathered. They followed the meal. They wouldn't sit and play on their Apple iStone Tablet. If they did, they'd starve to death.

So all the sugar that is consumed in the modern diet, which is bad enough, does not even burn due to sedentary lifestyles. This means energy spikes and shocks, and related health problems such as diabetes and blood pressure problems.

One of the great myths that the Paleo diet has helped dispel is the old-fashioned notion that eating fat makes you fat.

This was a big problem when the carbohydrate craze started in the eighties and everyone was obsessed with how many calories of fat they were eating. Almost all existing foods ended up with a low-fat or fat-free version. But most of that fat was replaced by sugar!

Fat is a crucial nutrient when it comes to our health. Dietary fat is necessary for an optimal, healthy and well-functioning body. It's all the chemicals, preservatives and sugar added to our diets that lead to weight gain, health problems, energy problems and more.

What fats should I eat if I want to be much healthier?

The first point to keep in mind is that not all fats are equal. The second point worth remembering is that you don't get fat from eating fat. In fact, you should consume the right fats for good health. Fats make you feel happy and give you a number of benefits such as reducing your risk of cancer, boosting your immune system, and even helping you lose weight.

Yes! You need to eat fat to lose fat... but you must eat the right fats.

The problem these days is that most people are consuming unhealthy fats that come from hydrogenated oils. Many people are unaware of how unhealthy the vegetable oils they consume are. The oils are marketed as healthy and are made from natural foods such as soybeans, corn, etc..

In fact, oils that have been refined or hydrogenated are extremely bad for the human body and cause many health problems.

The paleo diet uses oils in their natural state. The oils are not bleached or subjected to chemical processes that make them harmful. The fats used in the paleo diet are not only safe but extremely beneficial to the body.

Because the diet is heavy on meat, you will get a good portion of animal fats in your diet. People on paleo diets are encouraged to get grass-fed meats because even the food commercial companies feed their livestock is harmful. Eating grass-fed meats will ensure that no adverse effects are transmitted to you.

Animal fats are perfectly fine. Our ancestors ate a lot of meat and our bodies have evolved over time to eat meat and handle animal fat. Rest assured that your cholesterol level will not skyrocket. Studies have shown that dietary cholesterol does not cause high cholesterol in humans.

The Real Causes of High Cholesterol

Hydrogenated oils are sold on supermarket shelves. Unhealthy fats found in cookies, junk food, fast food, etc. These are what cause unhealthy cholesterol levels. Don't worry! Since the paleo diet doesn't allow the consumption of these horrible items, you're safe.

Coconut oil is the preferred oil in the Paleo diet. Just as olive oil is a staple food in the Mediterranean diet, coconut oil is the staple oil in the Paleo diet. It contains more than 90% saturated fat and every bit is good for you. Coconut oil is stable at room temperature and can be used for cooking. Contains lauric acid that is easily digested and helps strengthen the immune system.

Another healthy fat observed in the paleo diet is olive oil. This is a very healthy oil and helps balance the omega-3 and omega-6 fatty acids in the body. This will lubricate your joints and prevent inflammation in the body.

Butter and ghee are other fats that are also used to prepare paleo dishes. Many paddle dieters stir their eggs in the morning with melted butter.

Butter is not a strictly paleo ingredient, but it has many health benefits. So, if you're willing to be a little lax, you can include butter as part of your diet. It has many benefits.

These are just some of the fats in the paleo diet. There are other fats like avocado oil, etc. The point you should take from this article is that the fats in the paleo diet are perfectly healthy.

You should be more concerned with normal food that is sold commercially. These are the biggest culprits for most of society's health problems these days. Avoid these unhealthy products and go paleo. It really is a change of life.

The Paleo diet is known as the "caveman" diet because it is basically the diet you are asked to eat. Paleo's diet consists mainly of meat, fish, turkey, chicken, fruits, vegetables and nuts.

In general, Eating Paleo eliminates the negative aspects of the modern diet, such as sugar, trans fats and preservatives, while nourishing your body with vitamins, minerals, proteins and healthy fats such as essential fatty acids. Essential as your body needs them! Do you understand?

Well, that's a basic summary of what the Paleo diet is, in the next part we're going to look at going to organic farming and after that we're going to look at Paleo approved foods.

The importance of 100% organic food

Part of being an informed and conscientious consumer is being aware of the foods you buy and their health benefits and drawbacks, especially if you are thinking about adopting the Paleo way of eating.

Buzzwords circulate in the world of healthy eating so often that it is difficult to keep track of what is what and why, and "organic" is certainly no exception.

Walk into your typical daily grocery store and you will most likely run into some aisles labeled "healthy food aisle" or "organic aisle". Sounds pretty good, doesn't it?

The shelves are full of items labeled "natural," "raw," "sprouted," and "organic. Prices are a little high, but that's the price you pay for health, isn't it?

The term organic refers to the way agricultural products are grown, cultivated, handled and processed. The use of natural fertilizers over chemicals and natural insecticides over synthetics are two ways in which food can be grown and processed to be considered organic. Meat that is considered organic comes from animals that were given organic food and does not contain antibiotics, growth hormones, or medications.

Labelling of organic food

- 100% organic - completely organic or made from all organic ingredients
- Organic - at least 95% organic ingredients
- Made with organic ingredients - 70% or more organic ingredients

It is important to consider the value of buying a particular item in an organic variety. Just because organic costs are higher doesn't necessarily mean it's worth it.

Organic.org has a list of foods they call the "dirty dozen," which contain those that have the highest level of pesticides and are therefore best purchased organic.

There is also a list of a dozen foods that you can buy inorganically ("less contaminated"). This guide is a great reference for your trips to the grocery store.

> ***Adding organic foods to your paleolithic diet***

Now that you understand what organic means, what are some of the reasons why you should start adding organic foods to your grocery shopping if you follow a Paleo diet?

- More Nutritious - Vitamins, Minerals, Antioxidants, Flavonoids
- Safer - No pesticides, usually no GMOs
- Pure - No flavor enhancers, preservatives, contaminants

While many argue that the price of organic food makes it impossible to pay, there are ways to make it fit your budget.

- Shop at local farmers' markets
- Join an organic cooperative
- Buy directly from farmers
- Wholesale Purchase
- Grow your own
- Online Shop

Those who are fans of organic foods believe that it is healthier and safer to consume than non-organic foods when following the Paleo diet. On the other hand, some argue that there is no way to ensure that what you are buying is truly organic, the main factor is the consumption of these over-processed foods.

If you want to be healthy... You must consume this...

Foods you can eat: (we'll cover this in a little more detail below)

- Butter
- Eggs
- Fish and shellfish
- Fruit
- Herbs and spices
- Meat
- Natural oils (avocado, coconut, olive)
- Nuts (Seeds)
- Vegetables

> ***Foods that you should never eat (or at least reduce their consumption)***

Grains, grains, grains (barley, rye, wheat) - Among other things contain gluten. Avoiding grains means not eating bread or pasta.

Sugars (includes high fructose corn syrup) - No soft drinks, fruit drinks, ice cream, cakes, sweets, etc. Sugars can promote weight gain, cause diabetes, energy collisions and blood pressure problems, among other health problems.

Legumes - This means there are no beans or lentils.

Dairy - Stay away from all low-fat dairy products. If you don't have trouble digesting dairy products, it may be okay to consume some high-fat dairy products, such as whole raw milk and certain cheeses, but only in small amounts.

Hydrogenated vegetable oils (canola, corn, cottonseed, soybean, sunflower, etc.) - These oils cause unhealthy levels of inflammation. And remember the essential fatty acids mentioned above? One of the biggest problems today is our unbalanced intake of Omega-6 fatty acids compared to Omega-3s. An important factor in this unbalanced intake is the high levels of Omega-6 fatty acids in these oils.

Margarine - margarine was created as a "healthy" alternative to butter. Turns out butter is the healthiest choice. Most margarine contains high levels of deadly trans fats.

Artificial sweeteners - things like acesulfame potassium, aspartame, saccharin and sucralose should be avoided in the Paleo diet.

   Obesity is an epidemic and many, many health problems have been linked to obesity. Obesity has been linked to diets high in processed foods, high in processed carbohydrates, and excessive intake of sugar. Potential health problems include heart disease, type 2 diabetes, cancer, and stroke.

Approved foods

Do you remember the above list of approved foods? We're talking burgers, steak, pork, bison, lamb, duck, turkey, chicken and more! Bacon, baby! The world is better with bacon!

Weed-fed if you can. After all, meat with a lot of added chemicals frustrates the purpose of the Paleo diet, don't you think?

Seafood includes fish such as salmon, trout, shrimp, a variety of seafood, haddock and much more.

You can eat lots of vegetables like carrots, broccoli, kale and tomato, as well as onions and peppers.

Sweet potatoes, sweet potatoes, sweet potatoes and baked potatoes are on the list of foods approved by Paleo. This includes turnips as well.

Yes to eggs too - boiled hard, boiled soft, scrambled, tortilla (just add some of those vegetables and even some from the meat list, if that's what you enjoy.

The nuts and approved seeds you can eat are almonds, walnuts, sunflower seeds, pumpkin seeds, hazelnuts, chia seeds and macadamia nuts as well.

A wide variety of fruits can be eaten when you go to Paleo. In this list there are all kinds of berries (strawberries, blueberries, blackberries, etc.), apples, oranges, mangoes and pears. This also includes avocados, which is a fantastic source of the vitamins, minerals and healthy fats your body needs.

Oils are an important part of the Paleo diet and include the olive, coconut and avocado mentioned above.

Finally, we have our herbs and spices. There is something here for everyone to spice up their food: sea salt, garlic, turmeric, mint, basil, rosemary and many others can be part of your daily diet.

In the Paleo diet or in the "Caveman" diet you will find slightly different approved foods. Some will tell you that it is okay to consume certain things in limited amounts. This includes red wine (science says red wine has a variety of health benefits), hot chocolate with dark chocolate, and certain teas, such as green tea, which is full of powerful antioxidants that have many health benefits.

Hardcore Paleo enthusiasts will tell you to go to organic farming as often as possible, eat only grass-fed meat and eat sustainable wild caught fish. If you can do this, great, but if you can't, don't let that stop you.

Following the Paleo diet will do wonders for you, even if you don't go to organic hardcore all the way. Do what you can.

What exercises to do during the paleolithic diet?

Exercise and nutrition go hand in hand. If you are going to embrace the Paleo lifestyle, you really should consider an exercise regimen as well. It doesn't have to be crazy, like a weight training program from a professional bodybuilder or the training of a high level athlete.

In fact, if all you can gather is a 30-minute walk every day, that's a big problem. One of the biggest problems of modern life is how sedentary we are today. Many people sit at a desk all day and then sit on the couch at night, usually with a smartphone, tablet or lap top, participating in social media sites.

So if you can walk every day for half an hour, good for you! Keep it up!

If you want a little more but are one of those people you REALLY struggle with to maintain your workouts, forget about the complicated multiple exercise programs.

Start by focusing on making exercises a habit so that they become part of your life routine. And the easiest way to do this is not just to exercise first thing in the morning, but to make exercise incredibly simple.

How do you make it so simple that you never skip a workout? Easy! As soon as you get out of bed, start exercising! This can be as simple as an exercise.

Here are a few examples. (See

demonstrations of exercises in Youtube if you are not sure)

If you can't take 50 straight breaks, take breaks when you need to and keep a record of how long it takes to complete the 50 and try to beat that amount the next time you do. Or, invest it and do it.

body weight is squatted for 7 minutes, resting when necessary and keeping a record of how many times you squat. Next time, try to do more in those 7 minutes.

You could do a different exercise each day for a week and then repeat it.

Maybe like this:

✓ Monday: Squatting body weight
✓ Tuesday: Push Ups
✓ Wednesday: Burpees
✓ Thursday: Jumps
✓ Friday: more jumps
✓ Saturday: Jump rope
✓ Sunday: Sunday rest

Modify the exercises to suit your needs. If you have knee problems or are severely overweight or out of shape, burpees and jumps may not be for you. That's very good. Do normal squats instead of bubbles. Make regular jumps instead of jumps.

Isn't she strong enough for the push-ups? Do it from your knees. Or do it on a wall, with your feet a few feet away, so you have to lean on the wall.

If push-ups are too easy, make a more difficult version, such as explosive push-ups, gonorrhea push-ups, or spider push-ups.

Once you've done it for a few weeks and exercise becomes normal in the morning, you can start doing multiple exercise routines.

Another option would be to make an appointment with yourself. Instead of having a workout scheduled for Tuesday, you should have an exercise appointment with yourself on Tuesday at 6 pm. You'll be much more likely to keep this commitment

Is the Palaeolithic diet suitable for my family?

If you are someone who is thinking about starting a Paleo eating plan and would like the whole family to join in the fun, but you don't know if it's the right thing to do or not, then you're not alone.

This question has been asked many times and in this chapter we will try to navigate through it.

First, before you approach your family and try to convince them to follow a paleo diet, there are a few things to keep in mind. First of all, as we have said, the paleo diet is not an easy diet. There are many restrictions such as not consuming sugar, processed foods, artificial additives, etc.

Secondly, it's not just a diet. It's all a lifestyle change. You won't be able to go to a party or meeting and eat what you want because there aren't many people who prepare the food according to the requirements of the paleo. Even restaurants and expensive meals; establishments will not be able to prepare food palaeographically. That basically means you'll have to bring your own food to a party.

Third, most comfort foods are excluded from the Paleo diet simply because they contain sugar, dairy products, or some ingredient that is not allowed in the Paleo diet.

So how are you going to convince your spouse and children to stop eating their favorite foods and eat like cavemen?

The process itself may look like you are in a UN convention trying to get opposing countries to sign a multilateral agreement.

The best way to do this would be to do it in stages. Don't try to move from zero to a hero paleo overnight. Yes, it's beneficial and yes, it's an excellent idea... but you'll have to give your family time to adapt, adapt and assimilate.

In the early stages, make a meal a paleo meal. Could be breakfast. Discard sugary cereals and milk. Replace with bacon fried in coconut oil, scrambled eggs and a glass of fresh fruit juice. Get a recipe book full of delicious recipes and tempt your family members with tasty paleo foods.

The key is to make them feel like they're not sacrificing delicious food for a paleo diet. Your excitement and interest, however contagious, may not be enough to convince your family to stay out of that tub of macadamia nut ice cream.

Also, try not to lecture too much and don't stand on a palace pedestal and shake your head at your poor food choices. Do tolerance exercises and slowly put them by your side.

Of course, your family can say, "Yes! Let's do the paleo diet and eat veal liver tonight".... very unlikely, but if this happens, good for you.

Otherwise, follow the advice above.

It is a fantastic idea to get your family on the paleo diet because it is very healthy. You will be less prone to obesity, allergies, aches and pains, etc. In the long run, your whole family will benefit from the paleo diet.

Therefore, it is worth pursuing and persuading him. Have tolerance or your spouse can divorce you and allow you to have full custody of the chicken legs and bison tail that are happily sitting in the freezer.

The key to convincing them will be to become an excellent cook. Invest in a good paleo recipe book and perfect your culinary skills. Concentrate on the desserts. Most people find it extremely difficult to stop eating sweet foods.

Do not use the Paleo diet as a crutch for

cooking unpleasant dishes. It is perfectly possible to prepare delicious paleo dishes. Once you can do that, it's half the battle won.

Work on yourself.... then work on your family. There are many families in the paleolithic diet. This objective is within reach

Conclusion

Congratulations on reaching the end of this guide to the Palaeolithic Diet.

You'll be surprised to learn that most people who start something never complete it. If you've come this far, you're definitely interested in Paleo's way of eating and all the benefits it offers.

The best thing you can do is get authorization from your doctor and start a Paleo program.

Take your time and progress at your own pace. This isn't a race. The more you do it, the better you'll do it and the healthier you'll be. It's all a matter of time and practice.

In this last part we will see the practical steps to start a Paleo lifestyle from today.

Understand what you should and shouldn't do to eat and what you shouldn't eat:

- *Eat:* Nuts, vegetables, fruits, eggs, organic and grass meats, healthy oils (coconut, avocado, olive, etc.), fish and seafood.

- *Don't eat:* Processed foods, dairy foods (butter, yogurt, cheese, milk), cereal grains, legumes (beans, peas), peanuts and peanut butter, refined sugar, potatoes, refined vegetable oils, candy, artificial sweeteners, starchy vegetables (potatoes, yams, etc.).

Do it in the long run:

Lasting results happen when you cling to something permanently. That doesn't mean that once in a while you don't find yourself drinking a cup of milk with an Oreo. But getting into a diet change with the mentality that the changes are permanent and lasting is the key to success.

Remember, this isn't a race. It may take some time to remember which foods to incorporate and which foods to give up.

Clean up your kitchen:

Let's face it. The box of cookies in your closet clearly won't fly into Paleo's world.

But if they're there, you'll probably eat them. The same goes for butter, peanuts, potatoes. To avoid temptations every time you open the cabinet door, you're going to have to throw away some of those things. Give it to a neighbor, a friend, or the local food bank.

Make sure you understand his reasoning:

We often read about a new diet or exercise and are so excited, we just want to dive in because the name sounds awesome! But to maintain our long-term motivation, it's important to understand why you're choosing to start something.

Are you diving at Paleo because your friend did it, because you want to feel better or because you want to lose weight? Whatever your reasoning, make sure it's one you really believe in.

➤ *Practicing forgiveness*

Apart from the fact that this is an impressive general rule for life, it reminds us that we are not perfect. From time to time we may want a treat (read: something not on Paleo's "eat" list).

Some people are allowed to treat from time to time-some do so on a scheduled basis, others as life gets rid of things. In spite of everything, don't punish yourself for "slipping." We're human after all!

➤ *Do your homework*

If you're a restaurant junkie and crying over the mere idea of giving up your

Friday night fun, wait a minute. Check the menus of the places you frequent and see how you can make food choices that meet Paleo's "requirements. Or, if there's a dish you can't live without, plan to cheat at the restaurant that serves it.

Making the decision to live a healthier life is impressive and admirable, whether Paleo ends up being the route for you or not. By eating the food our ancestors ate, instead of filling our stomachs with everything they carried, we can be sure that we are on a path of healthier and happier lives.

"Let food be your medicine, and medicine your food."

\- Hippocrates

Now yes, I wish you the best in your

results, and remember, everything is practical; theory without action is of no use to you. It brings everything you learn into real life.

A big hug, your friend, Jessy!

By the way, when you achieve your results little by little, I highly recommend you, if you want to learn much more about methods of losing weight, my book, on "HOW TO MAKE THE CETOGENIC DIET WITHOUT STOP EATING", is a book that I am sure will help you a lot on your way to "good health". Without further ado, you can find it in the Amazon search engine, like: "how to do the ketogenic diet without stopping eating" or looking for my name, like: "Jessy M. Brown"... Once again I wish you success in your results!